You get to have your *(high-fat/ low-carb)* cake and eat it too

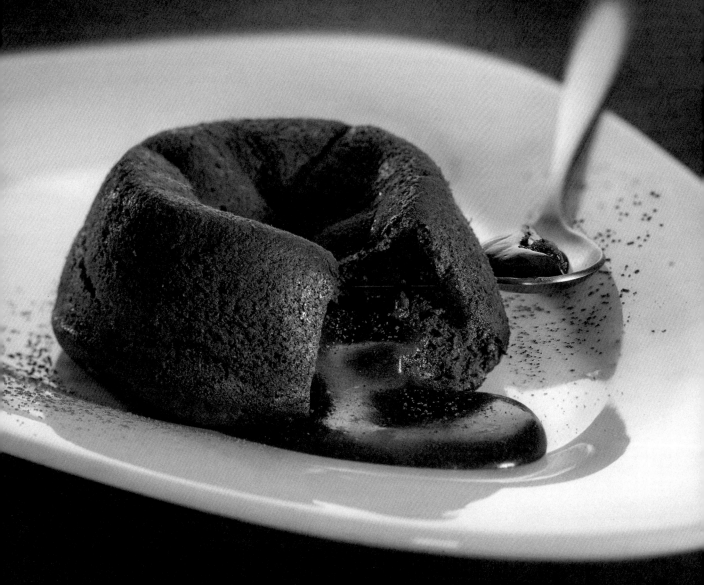

INTRODUCTION

It may seem strange that by eating "fat bombs," you can be healthier, but that is the promise and science behind a ketogenic diet. You can have your (high fat/low carb) cake and eat it too! By sticking to a low-carb diet, there are numerous benefits, including:

• Accelerated fat loss

• Lower cholesterol

• Lower blood sugar

• Increased energy and vitality

• Improved mental focus (ketogenic diets were initially used for epilepsy)

For me, the best part about high-fat foods is dessert. Particularly the new "category" of food invented just for the low-carb diet – the Fat Bomb.

To help you get the most out of this diet, below are 25 of the best high-fat/low-carb desserts available. I suggest trying at least one or two a week to help keep your motivation up. See them as a treat for being good throughout the week. The portioned treats are particularly great for this, such as cookies or truffles, as they can be stored away and enjoyed throughout the week.

I hope you enjoy the recipes and they help you on your journey to a healthier you.

Elizabeth

Keto Easy Meals Bonus Series

I am delighted you have chosen my book to help you start or continue on your keto journey.

Keto meals can be hard, complicated ingredients, long cooking times... to help you stay on the keto track, I am pleased to offer you three mini ebooks from my 'Keto Easy Meals Bonus Series', completely free of charge! These three mini ebooks cover how to make everything from easy breakfasts, to 6 ingredient dinners and meals using just one pot (less prep and washing up)!

Simply visit the link below to get your free copy of all three mini ebooks:

http://ketojane.com/mealsbonus

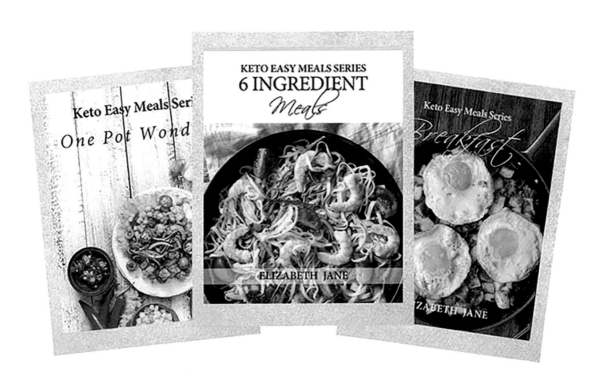

10
Chocolate Lava Cake (GF)

24
Chocolate Coconut Bites (GF)

11
Decadent Three-layered
Chocolate Cream Cake (GF)

25
Chocolate Walnut Fudge (GF)

13
Individual Strawberry
Cheesecakes (GF)

26
Easy Pecan and Maple Syrup Squares (GF)

14
Brownie Cheesecake Bars (GF)

27
Coconut Cream Brownies (GF)

15
Rich Chocolate Pudding (GF)

28
Mini Chocolate Avocado Tarts (GF

16
Fresh Strawberries with
Coconut Whip (GF, P)

29
Chocolate-drizzled
macaroons (GF)

17
Choco-nut Milkshake (GF)

30
Peanut Butter Cookies (GF)

18
Butter Pecan Ice cream (GF)

31
Dark Chocolate Tart (GF)

19
No-churn Blueberry Ice cream (GF)

32
Peanut Butter Cups (GF)

20
Carrot Cake with Cream Cheese Frosting (GF)

33
Mint Chocolate Chip Shake (GF, P)

21
Coconut Almond Cookies (GF)

34
Chocolate-covered
Almond (GF, P)

22
Peanut Butter and Jelly Cookies (GF)

35
No-flour Almond
Butter Cookies (GF, P)

25
Dark Chocolate Truffles (GF)

36
Snickerdoodle Bites (GF)

A Note About Sweeteners

Before we start talking about the different recipes, I'd like to take a moment to talk about the substitute sweeteners that we will be using.

Even people who are not on a ketogenic diet have come around to knowing the dangers of white sugar. Some people even refer to it as "white poison." Combine this with the rise in diabetes and weight-gain problems, sugar substitutes have spiraled up in popularity in the past few decades.

Now, there are many different sugar substitutes, and they come under various brand names, but some of the most common sugar substitutes include stevia and erythritol. However, I have also listed another natural sugar alternative, pure Grade B maple syrup. Keep in mind that when using the pure maple syrup, the carb count would be higher than using something like stevia.

Here is a little more information about stevia and erythritol if you decide to use these.

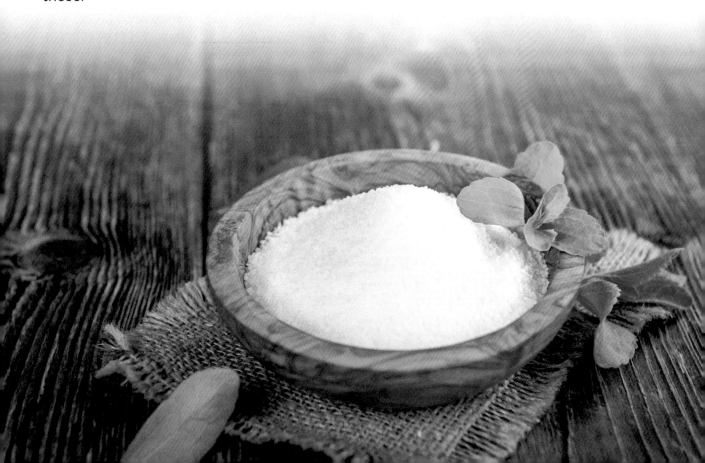

Stevia, or stevia extract as it should be called, is the extract of the stevia plant that occurs naturally. It is a zero-calorie sweetener so is perfect for our needs. In the market, it either comes in liquid or powder form. Both are fine. Powder form is more suited for use in cakes and baking while liquid is more suited for liquid-based recipes, such as smoothies. It is also recommended that you purchase a stevia that is free from any unnecessary added ingredients as some brands fill their products with other artificial ingredients that we want to avoid.

Erythritol, on the other hand, is a naturally occurring substance that is found in some fruits and cheeses. Like stevia, it is also calorie-free. However, one distinction between the two is that erythritol gives a glazed appearance to the dishes, making it perfect for icings, coatings and – yes –ice cream! Also, erythritol is a grain-to-grain sugar substitute, which means that one tablespoon of white sugar and one tablespoon of erythritol will give the same amount of sweetness, so using it is very easy.

Both are safe, heat-stable, and taste neutral. It is a good idea to have them both in your pantry. Preferably, you should have some liquid stevia and granulated erythritol on hand. However, if you have to choose, I'd suggest that you go with erythritol because it is more versatile and easier to use despite being a little pricier.

I hope that this cleared up the common confusion about non-calorie sweeteners.

So, let's get started.

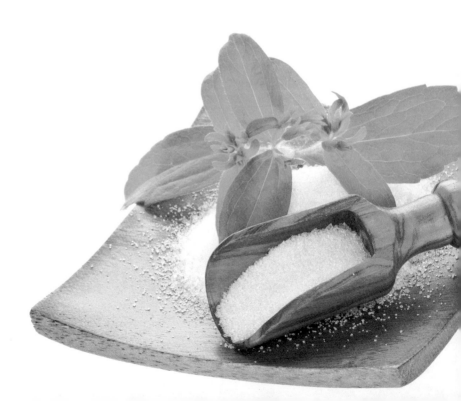

From the Author

This is a book focused on low-carb desserts, so you may be wondering what sets them apart from regularly enjoyed desserts and how they are made differently.

For starters, many of the recipes call for a sugar substitute, so sweeteners like stevia, erythritol, and even pure Grade B maple syrup are used in place of regular white sugar. This helps to cut the carb content especially if you are using stevia or erythritol. Many of the recipes also focus on using whole and natural ingredients, so you want to use foods like nut butters, coconut, and unsweetened dark chocolate instead of the processed versions you would find in store-bought dessert items.

In this book, you will find a variety of low-carb dessert options from cakes and cookies to ice cream and fudge. I hope that you enjoy them as much as I enjoyed preparing this book for you! Life is too short not to enjoy a treat every once in a while, and this is especially true when you are giving these lower-carb options a try.

Lastly, if you would be kind enough to leave an honest review, it would be most appreciated.

Please visit the below link.

http://ketojane.com/dessertreview

Once again, thank you for downloading and good luck.

Elizabeth Jane

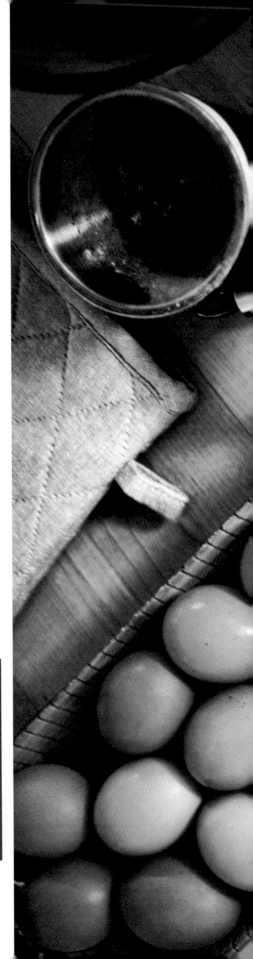

Dietary Labels

Within this book, you will notice that there are dietary labels. These will indicate whether a recipe is gluten-free or paleo. Please note that many recipes can be made dairy-free by removing the added cheese or by substituting the milk or cream for coconut milk. Each recipe will also be labeled if it is gluten-free. Although the majority of the recipes are gluten-free, variations in certain product ingredients mean that not all recipes will be marked gluten-free. If you wish to make all recipes gluten-free, be sure to check the food label on the ingredients you buy. You will also notice that if a recipe is not labeled as paleo-friendly that I have made some suggestions on how to make most of the recipes paleo-friendly by swapping out certain ingredients.

GF: Gluten-free

P: Paleo

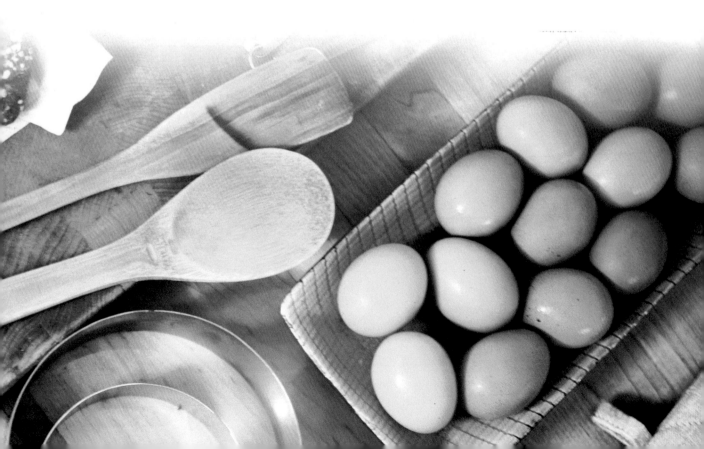

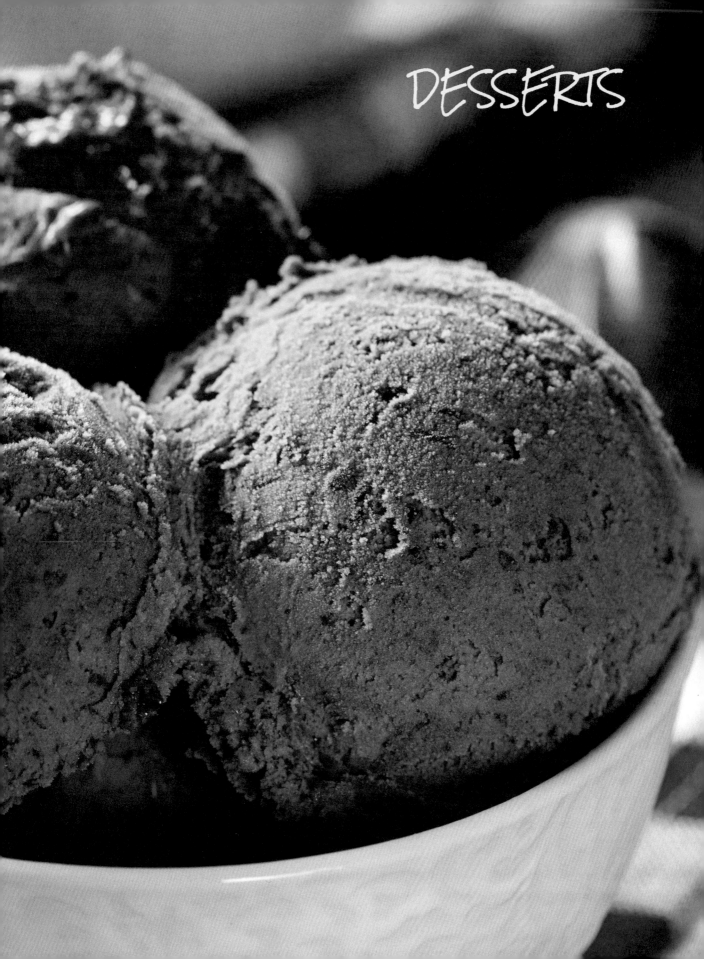

DESSERTS

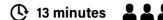 **10 minutes**   **13 minutes**

CHOCOLATE LAVA CAKE (GF)

INGREDIENTS

» ½ cup raw unsweetened cocoa powder
» ¼ cup butter, melted
» 4 eggs
» ¼ cup sugar-free and gluten-free chocolate sauce
» ½ teaspoon ground cinnamon
» ½ teaspoon sea salt
» 1 teaspoon pure vanilla extract
» ¼ cup raw stevia

DIRECTIONS

1. Pour 1 tablespoon of chocolate sauce into 4 cavities of an ice cube tray and freeze it.
2. Preheat oven to 350°F. Prepare 4 ramekins by greasing with oil or butter.
3. Whisk together the cocoa powder, stevia, cinnamon, and sea salt in a small bowl.
4. Whisk in the eggs, one at a time.
5. Add the melted butter and vanilla extract. Stir until well combined.
6. Fill each prepared ramekin halfway with the mixture.
7. Remove the chocolate sauce from the freezer and place one in each of the ramekins.
8. Cover the chocolate with the remaining cake batter.
9. Bake for 13 to 14 minutes or until just set. Transfer from the oven to a wire rack and allow to cool for 5 minutes.
10. Carefully remove the cakes from the ramekins.
11. Enjoy your tasty and healthy chocolate lava cake by cutting into its molten center.

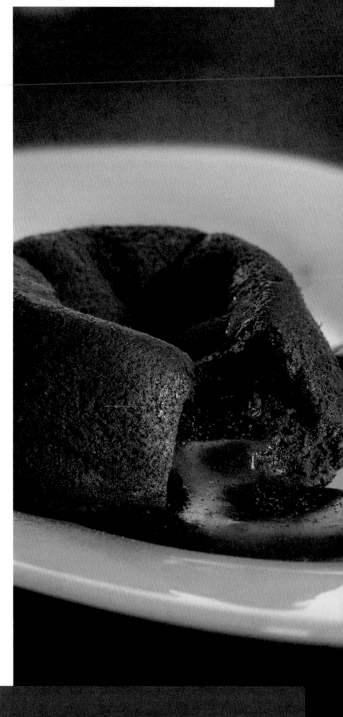

NUTRITION FACTS (PER SERVING)

Total Carbohydrates: 6g	Dietary Fiber: 3g	Net Carbs: 3g
Protein: 8g	Total Fat: 17g	Calories: 189

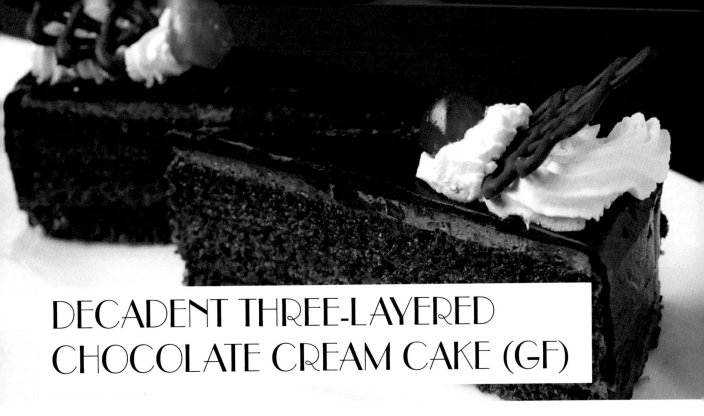

DECADENT THREE-LAYERED CHOCOLATE CREAM CAKE (GF)

 30 minutes   🕐 **60 minutes**   👤 **x8**

INGREDIENTS

» 4 ounces unsweetened chocolate
» ½ cup (1 stick) butter
» 1 ½ cups powdered sweetener, divided
» 3 eggs
» ½ cup + 8 tablespoons raw unsweetened cocoa powder
» 1 vanilla pod
» Pinch of sea salt
» 1 cup whipping cream
» Coconut whipped cream
» 1 can coconut milk, refrigerated overnight

DIRECTIONS

1. Preheat the oven to 325°F. Spray a little cooking oil into a pan smaller than 8 inches.
2. Combine the chocolate and butter in a double boiler and melt them together. Stir in ½ cup of sweetener and keep on stirring over low heat until everything is well combined. Remove from heat and let cool a little bit.
3. Separate the eggs, and beat the whites until stiff peaks form. Add ¼ cup of sweetener little by little.

4. Whisk the yolks together with another ¼ cup of sweetener. Add the chocolate mixture to the yolks and stir well. Mix in ½ cup cocoa, and then scrape the vanilla seeds from the pod and add to the mixture along with salt.
5. Fold in egg whites slowly to the chocolate mixture, but do not over mix.
6. Cook in the preheated oven for 1 hour or until a toothpick comes out clean. Let it cool completely and then remove from the pan.

Cream:

1. To prepare the 3 types of filling, beat the whipping cream for about 6-7 minutes until it gets very thick. Slowly add ½ cup of sweetener.
2. Divide the cream into halves and place one half in a bowl. Divide the remaining cream into halves again and place in other 2 separate bowls. You will have 3 bowls, one with ½ of the cream and two with ¼ of the cream.
3. Take a bowl with ¼ cream, add 1 tablespoon of cocoa powder and mix well. This will be the lightest-colored cream.
4. Add ½ the cream to the bowl, add 3 tablespoons of cocoa powder. Mix until well distributed. This will be the middle-colored cream.
5. Add 3–4 tablespoons of cocoa powder to the last bowl with ¼ cream. This will be the darkest cream.

Assembling:

1. Slice the cake horizontally in 3 equal slices using a very sharp knife.
2. Place the bottom part on a serving plate and cover with the middle-colored cream. Repeat with the second layer.
3. Top with the third cake piece and spread the light-colored cream on top, followed by the darkest cream.
4. Cut in 8 slices and enjoy.

NUTRITION FACTS (PER SERVING)

Total Carbohydrates: 11g	Dietary Fiber: 6g	Net Carbs: 5g
Protein: 7g	Total Fat: 27g	Calories: 304

INDIVIDUAL STRAWBERRY CHEESECAKES (GF)

INGREDIENTS

Crust

» ½ cup almond flour

» 3 tablespoons butter, melted (use coconut oil for a paleo version)

» ¼ cup sugar substitute (use pure Grade B maple syrup for a paleo version)

Filling

» 6 strawberries

» 3 tablespoons sugar substitute (use pure Grade B maple syrup for a paleo version)

» 8 ounces cream cheese (use full-fat unsweetened coconut cream for a paleo version)

» ⅓ cup sour cream (eliminate for a paleo version)

» ½ teaspoon pure vanilla extract

» 4 strawberries, quartered (for garnish)

» Fresh mint leaves (optional for garnish)

DIRECTIONS

1. To prepare the crust, place the almond flour, melted butter, and sugar substitute in a medium bowl and mix well to combine.

2. Divide the mixture evenly into 4 small serving bowls or ramekins, lightly pressing with your hands.

3. To prepare the filling, puree the strawberries in a food processor.

4. Add the sugar substitute, vanilla extract, cream cheese, and sour cream. Blend until smooth and creamy.

5. Spoon the mixture over the crust and chill for at least 1 hour.

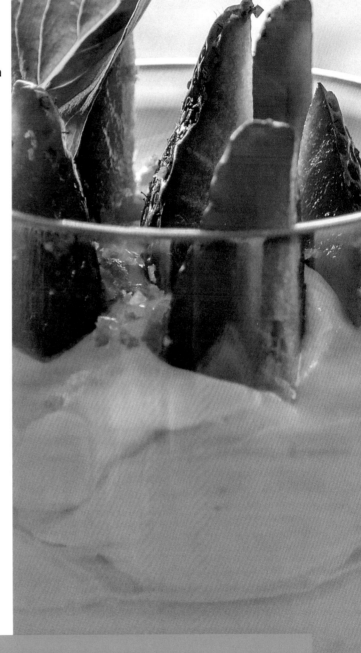

NUTRITION FACTS (PER SERVING)

Total Carbohydrates: 12g	Dietary Fiber: 3g	Net Carbs: 9g
Protein: 8g	Total Fat: 47g	Calories: 489

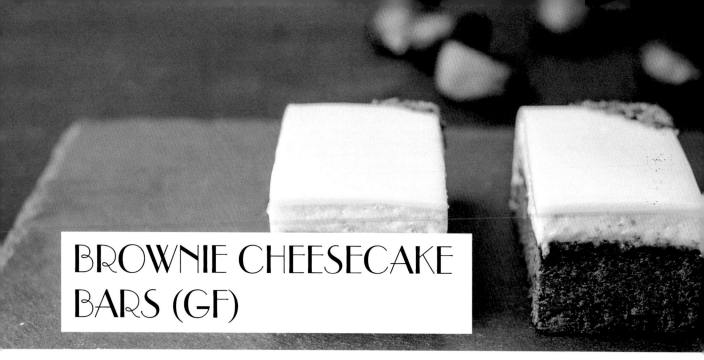

BROWNIE CHEESECAKE BARS (GF)

🥄 **50 minutes**   🕐 **55 minutes**   👤 **x6**

INGREDIENTS

Brownie layer

» 2 ounces bittersweet chocolate, chopped

» ½ cup butter, softened

» ⅓ cup raw unsweetened cocoa powder

» ½ cup almond flour

» 2 large eggs

» ½ cup sugar substitute

» ½ teaspoon pure vanilla extract

» ¼ teaspoon salt

Cheesecake layer

» 2 large eggs

» 16 ounces cream cheese, softened

» ⅓ cup sugar substitute

» ¼ cup heavy cream

» ½ teaspoon pure vanilla extract

DIRECTIONS

1. Preheat oven to 325°F.
2. Grease an 8x8 glass baking dish with butter or oil.
3. Melt the chocolate and butter together in a small saucepan over medium heat. Stir until well combined.
4. Whisk the almond flour, cocoa powder, and salt together in a small bowl.
5. Whisk the eggs, sugar substitute, and vanilla extract in a large bowl until frothy. Slowly whisk in the melted chocolate mixture.
6. Stir in the almond flour mixture and mix until smooth.
7. Pour into the prepared baking dish and bake for 20 minutes. Transfer to a wire rack and allow to cool.
8. For the cheesecake layer, mix together the cream cheese, eggs, sugar substitute, heavy cream, and vanilla extract with an electric mixer.
9. Reduce the oven heat to 300°F. Pour the batter over the baked brownies and return to the oven for 40 to 45 minutes or until set.
10. Remove from the oven and cool in the fridge for at least 2 hours prior to serving.

NUTRITION FACTS (PER SERVING)

Total Carbohydrates: 12g	Dietary Fiber: 3g	Net Carbs: 9g
Protein: 13g	Total Fat: 54g	Calories: 566

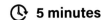
RICH CHOCOLATE PUDDING (GF)

INGREDIENTS

- » 2 cups coconut milk, canned
- » ¼ cup raw unsweetened cocoa powder
- » 1 tablespoon stevia
- » 2 tablespoons gelatin
- » 4 tablespoons water
- » ½ cup heavy whipping cream, beaten to stiff peaks
- » 1 ounce chopped bittersweet chocolate (optional for garnish)

DIRECTIONS

1. Heat the coconut milk, cocoa powder, and stevia in a small saucepan over medium heat. Stir until the cocoa powder and stevia have dissolved.
2. Mix the gelatin with the water and add to the saucepan. Stir until well combined.
3. Pour the mixture into 4 small ramekins or glasses.
4. Place the ramekins in the refrigerator for at least 1 hour.
5. Top with whipped cream, and chopped chocolate, if desired.

NUTRITION FACTS (PER SERVING)

Total Carbohydrates: 14g	Dietary Fiber: 5g	Net Carbs: 10g
Protein: 8g	Total Fat: 37g	Calories: 389

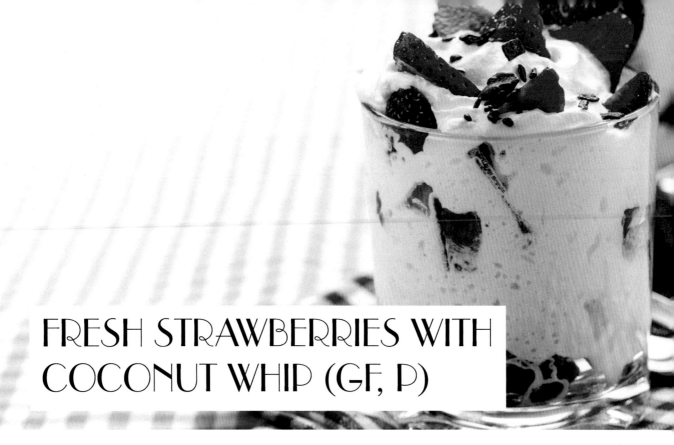

FRESH STRAWBERRIES WITH COCONUT WHIP (GF, P)

🥄 **5 minutes**   🕐 **3 minutes**   👤👤👤👤

INGREDIENTS

» 2 cans coconut cream, refrigerated
» 4 cups strawberries (can also use blueberries, blackberries, raspberries, or a combination)
» 1 ounce chopped unsweetened 70% or darker dark chocolate

DIRECTIONS

1. Scoop the solidified coconut cream (reserving the liquid in the bottom of the can for another use) into a large bowl and blend with a hand mixer on high for about 5 minutes or until stiff peaks form.
2. Slice the strawberries and arrange them in 4 small serving bowls.
3. Dollop the coconut whipped cream on top of the strawberries.
4. Garnish with chopped dark chocolate and additional berries.
5. Serve and enjoy!

NUTRITION FACTS (PER SERVING)

Total Carbohydrates: 15g	Dietary Fiber: 5g	Net Carbs: 10g
Protein: 4g	Total Fat: 31g	Calories: 342

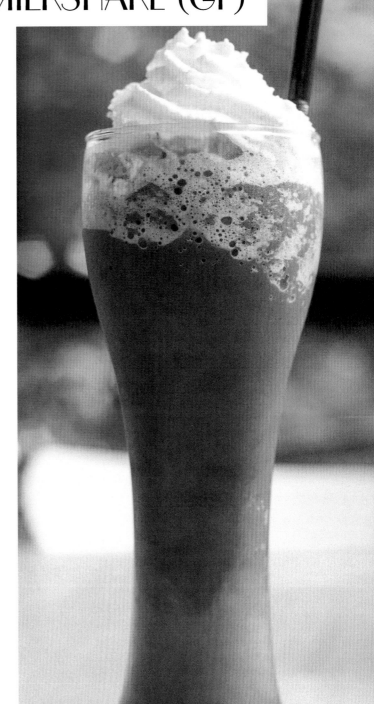

5 minutes   **0 minutes**

CHOCO-NUT MILKSHAKE (GF)

INGREDIENTS

» 2 cups unsweetened coconut, almond, or dairy-free milk of choice
» 1 banana, sliced and frozen
» ¼ cup unsweetened coconut flakes
» 1 cup ice cubes
» ¼ cup macadamia nuts, chopped
» 3 tablespoons sugar-free sweetener (use pure Grade B maple syrup for a paleo version)
» 2 tablespoons raw unsweetened cocoa powder
» Whipped coconut cream (optional for garnish)

DIRECTIONS

1. Place all ingredients into a blender and blend on high until smooth and creamy.
2. Divide evenly between 4 "mocktail" glasses and top with whipped coconut cream, if desired.
3. Add a cocktail umbrella and toasted coconut for added flair.
4. Enjoy your delicious choco-nut smoothie!

NUTRITION FACTS (PER SERVING)

Total Carbohydrates: 12g	Dietary Fiber: 4g	Net Carbs: 8g
Protein: 3g	Total Fat: 17g	Calories: 199

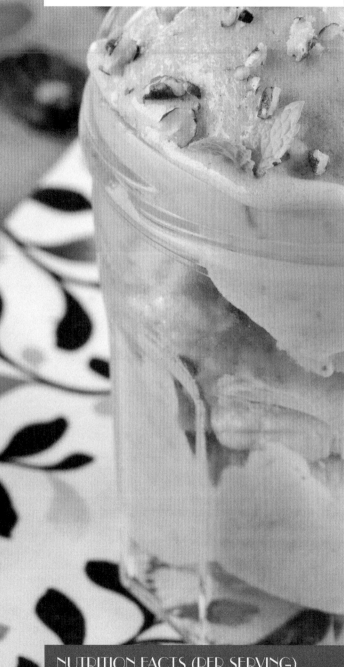

BUTTER PECAN ICE CREAM (GF)

INGREDIENTS

» ½ cup chopped pecans
» ⅛ teaspoon xanthan gum
» 2 egg yolks
» 1 teaspoon pure vanilla extract
» ¼ cup sugar substitute
» 2 tablespoons butter
» 1 cup heavy cream

DIRECTIONS

1. Melt the butter in a small saucepan over medium heat. Whisk the heavy cream into the butter after it has melted and become slightly brown.
2. Stir in the sugar substitute and mix until dissolved.
3. Add the xanthan gum and whisk until well combined. Transfer to a large, metal bowl and allow to cool.
4. Add the egg yolks slowly, one at a time, using a hand mixer.
5. Stir in the pecans and vanilla extract.
6. Place the bowl in the freezer for at least 4 hours, stirring well every hour.
7. Remove from the freezer and scoop into serving bowls.
8. Garnish with additional chopped pecans, if desired, and serve!

NUTRITION FACTS (PER SERVING)

Total Carbohydrates: 2g	Dietary Fiber: 1g	Net Carbs: 1g
Protein: 3g	Total Fat: 24g	Calories: 230

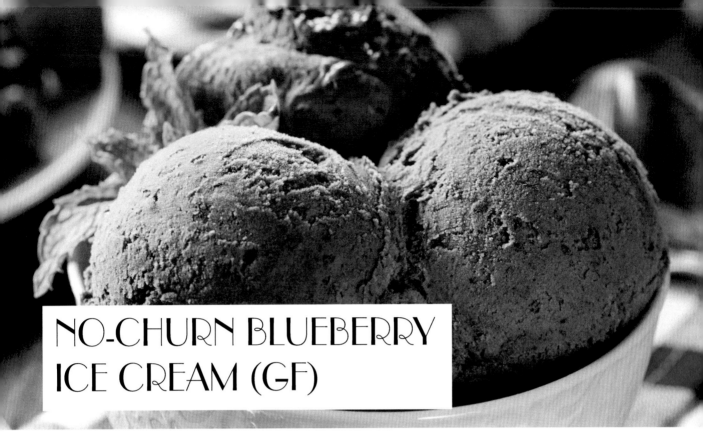

NO-CHURN BLUEBERRY ICE CREAM (GF)

 15 minutes   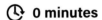 **0 minutes**

INGREDIENTS

- » ¼ cup crème fraîche or sour cream (be sure to check the label for GF labeling)
- » 1 cup heavy whipping cream
- » ¼ cup fresh blueberries
- » 1 egg yolk, beaten
- » 2 teaspoons pure vanilla extract

DIRECTIONS

1. Whip the crème fraîche with a hand mixer until frothy.
2. Whip the heavy cream in a separate bowl until soft peaks form.
3. Fold the crème fraîche into the whipped cream carefully.
4. Puree the blueberries in a food processor or blender until smooth.
5. Stir the blueberry puree, egg yolk, and vanilla extract into the whipped cream mixture. Mix until just combined.
6. Transfer mixture into a loaf pan and freeze for 2 hours, stirring well every 30 minutes.
7. Scoop into serving bowls and enjoy your fresh blueberry ice cream!

NUTRITION FACTS (PER SERVING)

Total Carbohydrates: 3g	Dietary Fiber: 0g	Net Carbs: 3g
Protein: 2g	Total Fat: 15g	Calories: 153

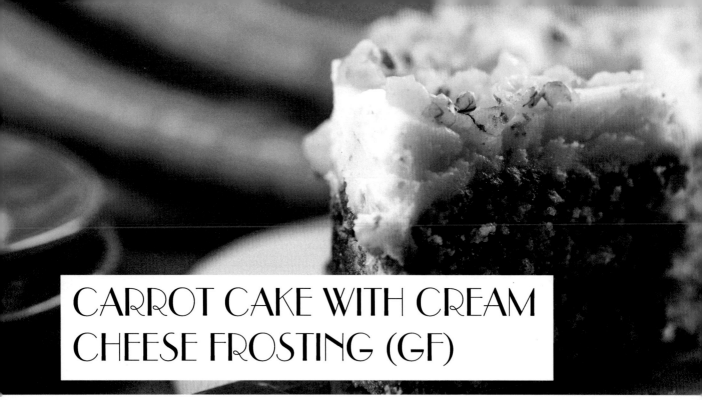

CARROT CAKE WITH CREAM CHEESE FROSTING (GF)

🥄 **15 minutes**   🕐 **30 minutes**   👤 **x6**

 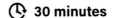

INGREDIENTS

Carrot cake

» 1½ cups carrots, grated finely

» ¾ cups sugar substitute

» ¼ cup brown sugar substitute

» ½ cup coconut oil, melted

» 2 large eggs

» ¼ cup flax meal

» ½ teaspoon baking soda

» ½ teaspoon ground cinnamon

» ¼ teaspoon ground nutmeg

» ¾ cup almond flour

Cream Cheese Frosting

» 8 ounces cream cheese, softened

» 2 tablespoons pure Grade B maple syrup

» ¼ teaspoon pure vanilla extract

» ¼ cup toasted walnuts, chopped (optional for garnish)

DIRECTIONS

1. Preheat oven to 350°F. Grease a 9-inch round cake pan with butter or oil.

2. Blend the sugars, coconut oil, and eggs together using a hand mixer.

3. Whisk the dry ingredients together in a separate bowl until well combined.

4. Add the dry ingredients slowly and keep blending until no lumps remain.

5. Stir in the grated carrots and pour into the prepared cake pan. Bake for 30 minutes or until a toothpick inserted comes out clean.

6. Remove from oven and allow to cool.

7. To prepare the frosting, beat the cream cheese, maple syrup, and vanilla extract until light and fluffy.

8. Top the cake with the frosting, sprinkle with toasted walnuts, slice, and serve!

NUTRITION FACTS (PER SERVING)

Total Carbohydrates: 14g	Dietary Fiber: 5g	Net Carbs: 9g
Protein: 11g	Total Fat: 45g	Calories: 479

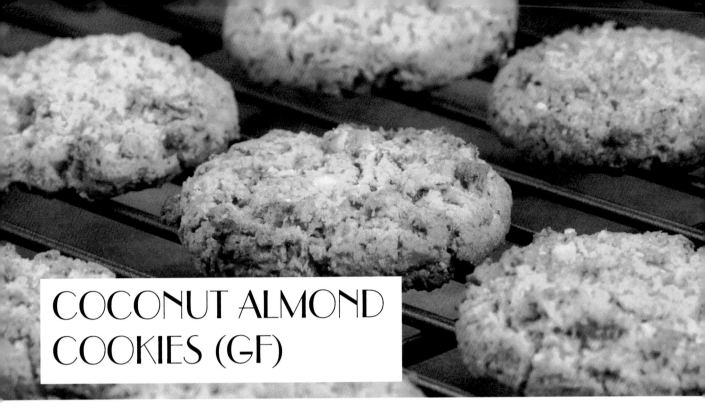

COCONUT ALMOND COOKIES (GF)

🥄 10 minutes   🕐 15 minutes   👤 x6

INGREDIENTS

- » 1¼ cups almond flour
- » ½ cup unsweetened, shredded coconut
- » 3 large eggs
- » 6 tablespoons butter, softened (use coconut oil for a paleo version)
- » ⅓ cup sugar substitute (use pure Grade B maple syrup for a paleo version)
- » 1 teaspoon almond extract
- » ¼ teaspoon ground cinnamon
- » ¼ teaspoon sea salt

DIRECTIONS

1. Preheat oven to 350°F. Prepare a metal baking sheet with parchment paper or non-stick spray.
2. Use a hand mixer to blend together the sugar substitute with the softened butter until smooth and creamy.
3. Add the eggs, one at a time, and mix until well combined.
4. Add the almond flour, almond extract, cinnamon, and salt with the mixer on low, mixing until just combined.
5. Stir in the shredded coconut.
6. Drop by the spoonful onto the baking sheet.
7. Bake for 12-15 minutes, until golden brown around the edges.
8. Remove from the oven and cool on a wire rack.

NUTRITION FACTS (PER SERVING)

Total Carbohydrates: 5g	Dietary Fiber: 3g	Net Carbs: 2g
Protein: 7g	Total Fat: 25g	Calories: 271

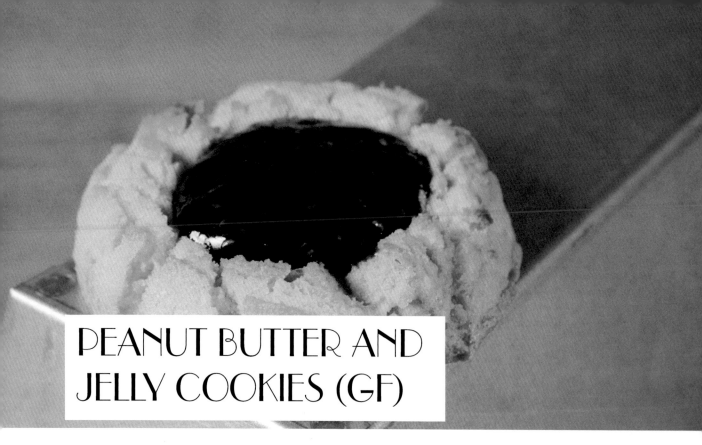

PEANUT BUTTER AND JELLY COOKIES (GF)

🥄 **10 minutes**   🕐 **12 minutes**   👤 **x6**

INGREDIENTS

- » ⅔ cup creamy peanut butter
- » ⅓ cup sugar-free strawberry preserves (be sure to check the label for GF labeling)
- » ⅓ cup almond flour
- » 1 egg
- » ½ cup sugar substitute
- » ¼ teaspoon pure vanilla extract
- » ¼ teaspoon baking powder
- » ¼ teaspoon sea salt

DIRECTIONS

1. Preheat oven to 350°F. Prepare a metal baking sheet with parchment paper or nonstick spray.
2. Beat the egg together with the peanut butter and sugar substitute in a large bowl until smooth and creamy. Add the almond flour, baking powder, salt, and vanilla extract. Mix well to form a dough.
3. Shape the mixture into small balls and arrange on the prepared baking sheet.
4. Make a small well in the middle of each cookie and fill with about 1 teaspoon of the preserves.
5. Bake for 10-12 minutes until the cookies are golden brown.
6. Cool on a wire rack and enjoy!

NUTRITION FACTS (PER SERVING)

Total Carbohydrates: 7g	**Dietary Fiber: 2g**	**Net Carbs: 5g**
Protein: 9g	**Total Fat: 18g**	**Calories: 209**

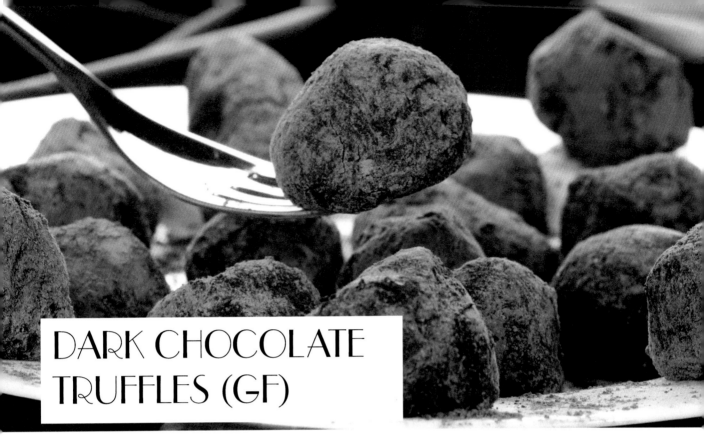

DARK CHOCOLATE TRUFFLES (GF)

🥄 **10 minutes**   🕐 **20 minutes**   👤 **x6**

INGREDIENTS

- » 4 ounces unsweetened dark chocolate (80% cocoa or higher)
- » 1 tablespoon raw unsweetened cocoa powder
- » 1 tablespoons pure Grade B maple syrup
- » 1½ tablespoons butter (use coconut oil for a paleo version)
- » ⅓ cup heavy cream (use full-fat unsweetened coconut cream for a paleo version)
- » ¼ teaspoon pure vanilla extract
- » ¼ teaspoon ground cinnamon
- » Pinch of sea salt

DIRECTIONS

1. Chop the dark chocolate finely.
2. Heat the heavy cream in a small saucepan over medium-low heat. Mix in the chopped chocolate and butter. Stir until melted and well combined.
3. Remove from heat and stir the vanilla extract, maple syrup, salt, and cinnamon.
4. Place mixture in the fridge for at least 2 hours.
5. Remove the mixture from the fridge once cooled and shape them into small balls using your palms.
6. Roll each ball in cocoa powder until coated fully.
7. Store in an airtight container in the fridge.

NUTRITION FACTS (PER SERVING)

Total Carbohydrates: 11g	Dietary Fiber: 1g	Net Carbs: 10g
Protein: 2g	Total Fat: 11g	Calories: 160

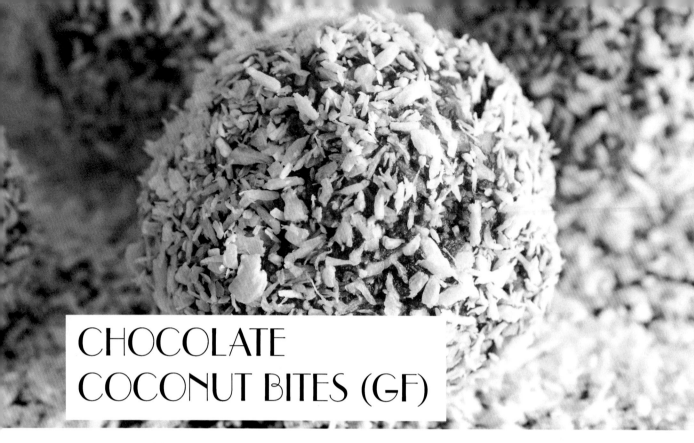

CHOCOLATE COCONUT BITES (GF)

🥄 5 minutes   🕐 7 minutes   👤 x6

INGREDIENTS

» 4 ounces unsweetened dark chocolate (80% cocoa or higher)
» ¼ cup unsweetened, shredded coconut
» 1 cup coconut flour
» 1 tablespoon chocolate protein powder (use a paleo-friendly version if you are following a paleo diet)
» 4 tablespoons coconut oil
» ⅓ cup heavy cream (use full-fat unsweetened coconut milk for a paleo version)

DIRECTIONS

1. Chop the dark chocolate into small pieces.
2. Heat the heavy cream in a small saucepan over medium-low heat. Add the chocolate and coconut oil and stir until melted and well combined.
3. Remove from heat and stir in the coconut flour and protein powder.
4. Place this mixture in the fridge for at least 2 hours.
5. Remove from the fridge once cooled and shape into small balls using your palms.
6. Roll each ball in the shredded coconut until coated fully.
7. Store in an airtight container in the fridge.

NUTRITION FACTS (PER SERVING)

Total Carbohydrates: 12g	Dietary Fiber: 3g	Net Carbs: 9g
Protein: 9g	Total Fat: 27g	Calories: 326

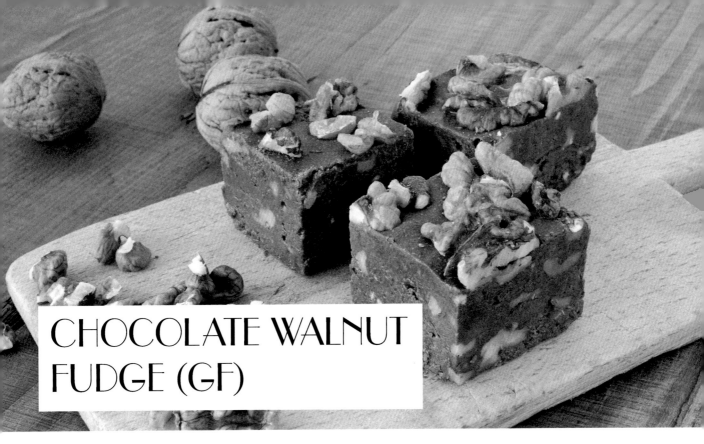

CHOCOLATE WALNUT FUDGE (GF)

🥄 **10 minutes**　　🕐 **5 minutes**　　👤👤👤👤

INGREDIENTS

» 2 tablespoons raw unsweetened cocoa powder
» 2 tablespoons sugar substitute (use pure Grade B maple syrup for a paleo version)
» 3 tablespoons coconut oil
» ¼ cup chopped walnuts
» ¼ cup heavy cream (use full-fat unsweetened coconut milk for a paleo version)
» 1 teaspoon pure vanilla extract

DIRECTIONS

1. Place the coconut oil in a metal bowl atop a pot of simmering water. Stir until melted.
2. Whisk in the cocoa powder and the sugar substitute.
3. Remove from heat and stir in the walnuts, heavy cream, and vanilla extract.
4. Stir until well combined and pour into chocolate molds or a square tray.
5. Let cool, then transfer to the fridge to harden.
6. Remove from the fridge and enjoy your delicious chocolate walnut fudge.

NUTRITION FACTS (PER SERVING)

Total Carbohydrates: 3g	Dietary Fiber: 1g	Net Carbs: 2g
Protein: 3g	Total Fat: 18g	Calories: 168

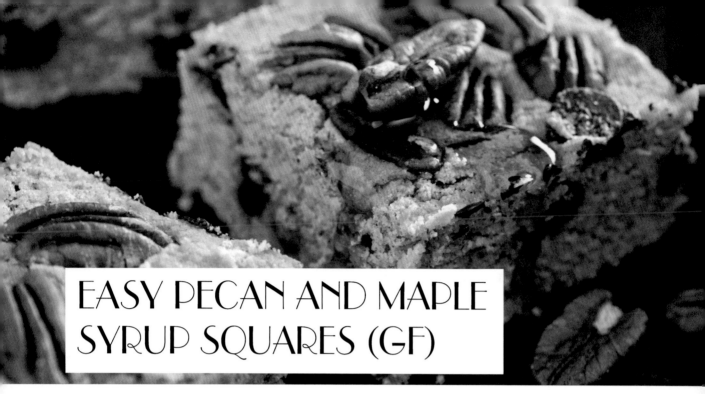

EASY PECAN AND MAPLE SYRUP SQUARES (GF)

🥄 **10 minutes**   🕐 **25 minutes**   👤 **x6**

INGREDIENTS

» 1 cup pecans (halved)
» 3 tablespoons pure Grade B maple syrup
» ½ cup almond flour
» ¼ cup flax meal
» ¼ cup unsweetened, shredded coconut
» ¼ cup coconut oil, melted
» 1 egg, beaten
» 2 tablespoons sugar substitute (use pure Grade B maple syrup for a paleo version)
» ⅓ cup sugar-free chocolate chips (optional) (skip for a paleo version)

DIRECTIONS

1. Preheat oven to 350°F degrees. Line a baking sheet with parchment paper. Place the pecans on the baking sheet and bake for 7 minutes, until toasted and fragrant.
2. Remove pecans from the oven and allow to cool. Chop the pecans once cooled, reserving a few halves for garnish.
3. Mix the flax meal, almond flour, chopped pecans, and shredded coconut together in a large bowl.
4. Stir in the maple syrup, coconut oil, egg, and sugar substitute. Mix well. Add the sugar-free chocolate chips, if using.
5. Transfer the dough into a 9-inch by 3-inch loaf pan that has been prepared with nonstick cooking spray.
6. Bake at 350°F for 20 minutes, or until a toothpick inserted comes out clean.
7. Remove from oven and allow to cool. Once cooled, place in the fridge for at least 2 hours.
8. Cut into squares and enjoy!

NUTRITION FACTS (PER SERVING)

Total Carbohydrates: 12g	**Dietary Fiber: 4g**	**Net Carbs: 8g**
Protein: 5g	**Total Fat: 21g**	**Calories: 233**

COCONUT CREAM BROWNIES (GF)

INGREDIENTS

» ¾ cup coconut butter, melted

» ⅓ cup coconut cream

» ¼ cup raw unsweetened cocoa powder

» ¼ cup coconut flour

» 2 tablespoons butter, melted (use coconut oil for a paleo version)

» ½ cup sugar substitute (use pure Grade B maple syrup for a paleo version)

» 1 egg

» 1 teaspoon pure vanilla extract

» ¼ teaspoon baking soda

» Pinch of sea salt

DIRECTIONS

1. Whisk the coconut flour, cocoa powder, sugar substitute, baking powder, and salt together in a large bowl.
2. Whisk the coconut butter, coconut cream and butter together in a separate bowl until well combined. Whisk in the egg and vanilla extract.
3. Stir the dry ingredients slowly into the wet ingredients and mix well.
4. Transfer the mixture into a 9-inch by 3-inch loaf pan that has been prepared with nonstick cooking spray.
5. Bake at 350°F for 20 minutes or until a toothpick inserted comes out clean.
6. Remove from the oven and cool to room temperature.
7. Cut into squares and enjoy!

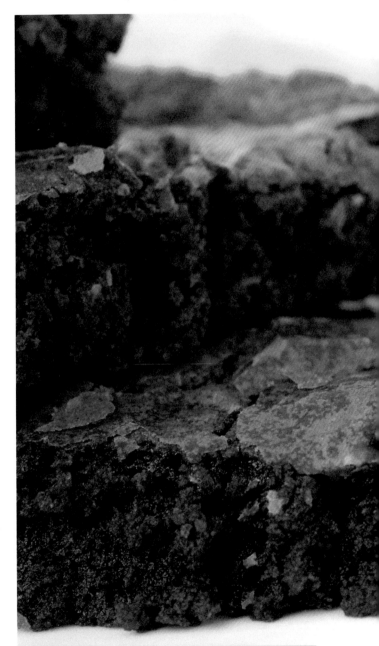

NUTRITION FACTS (PER SERVING)

Total Carbohydrates: 5g	Dietary Fiber: 3g	Net Carbs: 2g
Protein: 3g	Total Fat: 17g	Calories: 175

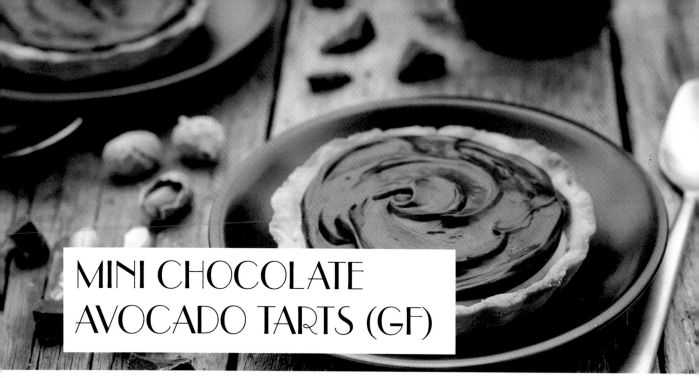

MINI CHOCOLATE AVOCADO TARTS (GF)

🥄 **15 minutes** 🕐 **8 minutes** 👤👤👤👤

INGREDIENTS

Tart crust

» 2 tablespoons almond flour
» 1 tablespoon sugar substitute (use pure Grade B maple syrup for a paleo version)
» 1 large egg white
» ¼ cup flax meal

Middle layer

» 4 tablespoons creamy peanut butter (use almond butter for a paleo version)
» 2 tablespoons butter (use coconut oil for a paleo version)

Top layer

» 1 medium avocado
» 4 tablespoons raw unsweetened cocoa powder
» ¼ cup sugar substitute (use pure Grade B maple syrup for a paleo version)
» 2 tablespoons heavy cream (use full-fat unsweetened coconut milk for a paleo version)
» ½ teaspoon pure vanilla extract

DIRECTIONS

1. Preheat the oven to 350°F.
2. Mix the almond flour, flax meal, 1 tablespoon of sugar substitute, and egg white together in a small bowl.
3. Press the mixture into 4 small tart tins. Bake for about 8 minutes, until golden. Remove from oven and allow to cool slightly.
4. Melt the peanut butter and butter in a small saucepan over medium-low heat and stir until well combined. Divide evenly between the baked tart shells. Transfer to fridge and allow to chill for 30 minutes.
5. Mix the avocado, cocoa powder, sugar substitute, heavy cream, and vanilla extract in a blender or food processor.
6. Remove the tarts from the fridge, top with the blended avocado mixture, and return to the fridge for at least 1 hour.
7. Serve and enjoy!

NUTRITION FACTS (PER SERVING)

Total Carbohydrates: 15g	Dietary Fiber:10g	Net Carbs: 5g
Protein: 11g	Total Fat: 33g	Calories: 367

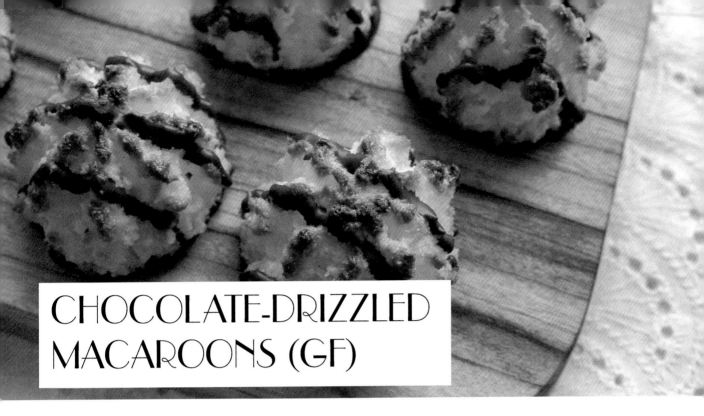

CHOCOLATE-DRIZZLED MACAROONS (GF)

10 minutes   **25 minutes**   👥👥👥

INGREDIENTS

- » 1 cup unsweetened shredded coconut
- » 2 ounces dark chocolate (80% cocoa or higher)
- » 2 large egg whites
- » ¼ cup sugar substitute (use pure Grade B maple syrup for a paleo version)
- » 2 tablespoons coconut oil
- » 1 teaspoon pure vanilla extract
- » Pinch of sea salt

DIRECTIONS

1. Preheat oven to 350°F. Prepare a metal baking sheet with parchment paper.
2. Spread the shredded coconut evenly onto the baking sheet and place in the oven to toast for 3-5 minutes or until light brown and fragrant.
3. Beat the egg whites with an electric mixer in a large mixing bowl. Add the sugar substitute slowly and continue mixing until stiff peaks form.
4. Stir in the toasted coconut, vanilla extract, and salt.
5. Line a baking sheet with parchment paper. Shape the mixture into balls using a small ice cream scoop or tablespoon and drop them onto the prepared baking sheet.
6. Bake for 15-18 minutes until golden brown. Remove from oven and cool on a wire rack.
7. Melt the dark chocolate together with the coconut oil in a small, microwave-safe bowl. Stir until well combined.
8. Drizzle the macaroons with the melted chocolate and enjoy!

NUTRITION FACTS (PER SERVING)

Total Carbohydrates: 8g	**Dietary Fiber: 2g**	**Net Carbs: 6g**
Protein: 3g	**Total Fat: 12g**	**Calories: 143**

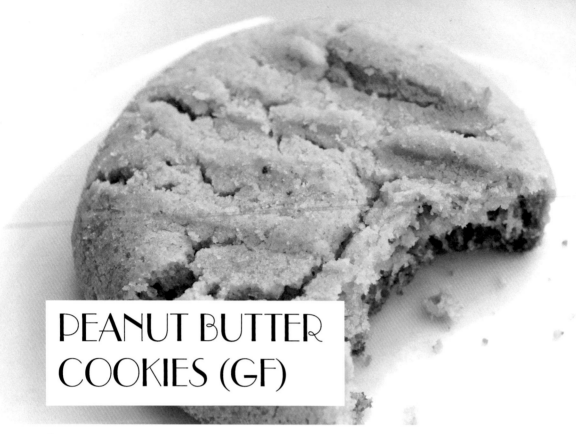

PEANUT BUTTER COOKIES (GF)

🥄 10 minutes　　🕐 15 minutes　　👤 x6

INGREDIENTS

- » ½ cup creamy peanut butter (use almond butter for a paleo version)
- » ½ cup coconut flour
- » ¼ cup sugar substitute (use pure Grade B maple syrup for a paleo version)
- » 1 egg
- » ¼ teaspoon pure vanilla extract
- » Pinch of sea salt

DIRECTIONS

1. Preheat oven to 350°F. Prepare a metal baking sheet with parchment paper or non-stick cooking spray.
2. Using an electric mixer, blend all ingredients together until a smooth dough forms.
3. Shape the dough into walnut-size balls and arrange on the prepared baking sheet.
4. Using a fork, make crisscross marks on top of the balls to form cookies and bake in the oven for 14-16 minutes, until golden brown.

NUTRITION FACTS (PER SERVING)

Total Carbohydrates: 5g	Dietary Fiber: 3g	Net Carbs: 2g
Protein: 7g	Total Fat: 14g	Calories: 160

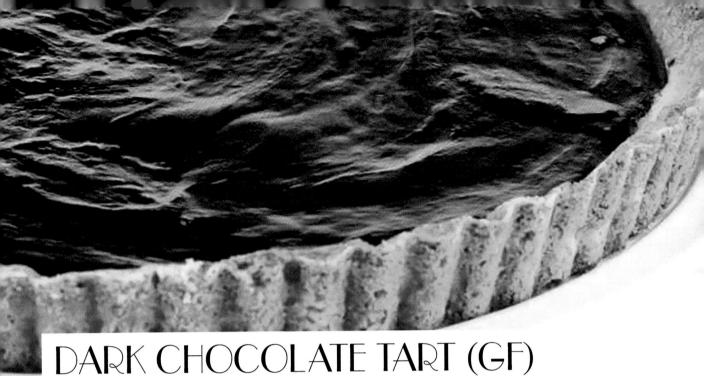

DARK CHOCOLATE TART (GF)

 20 minutes　🕐 **30 minutes**　👤👤👤👤

INGREDIENTS

Crust

» 1 cup coconut flour
» ¼ cup flaxseed meal
» 3 tablespoons sugar substitute (adjust according to taste)
» ½ cup butter
» 4 egg whites

Filling

» ½ cup raw unsweetened cocoa powder
» 1 cup heavy cream
» 2½ teaspoons gelatin powder
» ¼ cup sugar substitute (adjust according to taste)
» 1 teaspoon pure vanilla extract
» ¼ cup pistachios, sliced

DIRECTIONS

1. To prepare the crust: Preheat oven to 375°F. Prepare a small tart or pie pan with nonstick cooking spray.
2. Combine all of the crust ingredients in a food processor and pulse until well combined. Press the mixture into the prepared tart pan and bake for about 15 minutes. Remove from oven and allow to cool.
3. To prepare the filling: Combine all of the filling ingredients (reserving the pistachios) in a blender or food processor and blend until smooth and creamy.
4. Pour the mixture into the crust, cover with plastic wrap, and refrigerate for at least 2 hours.
5. Sprinkle with the reserved pistachios and serve!

ADDITIONAL TIP

* The time in fridge may vary, so watch the texture of the filling. It must be firm at the center.

NUTRITION FACTS (PER SERVING)

Total Carbohydrates: 13g	Dietary Fiber: 7g	Net Carbs: 6g
Protein: 13g	Total Fat: 46g	Calories: 490

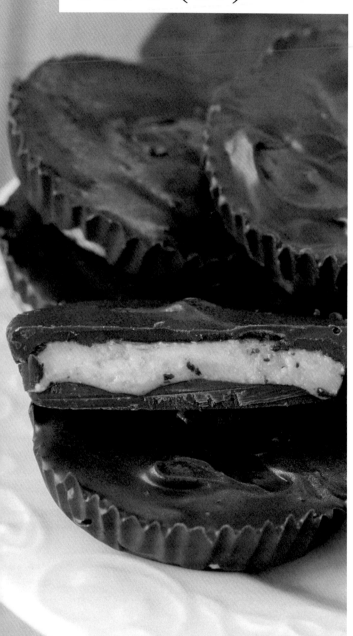

PEANUT BUTTER CUPS (GF)

INGREDIENTS

» ½ cup unsweetened dark chocolate baking chips
» ½ cup coconut oil
» ½ cup unsweetened peanut butter (use almond butter for a paleo version)
» 1 tsp. pure vanilla extract
» 2 tablespoons sugar substitute (use pure Grade B maple syrup for a paleo version)
» 1 teaspoons sea salt

DIRECTIONS

1. Line a mini muffin tin with muffins liners.
2. Add the dark chocolate, coconut oil, vanilla extract, sugar substitute, and sea salt to a stockpot and stir until completely melted.
3. Pour about 2 teaspoons of the chocolate mixture into the base of each lined muffin tin and top with a scoop of peanut butter. Set in the freezer for about 5 minutes to harden.
4. Remove the pan from the freezer and top with another 2 teaspoons or so of the melted chocolate mixture to completely cover the peanut butter.
5. Set the pan in the freezer and freeze for another 15-20 minutes or until the peanut butter cups are hardened.
6. Store leftovers in the fridge.

ADDITIONAL TIP

* The freezing times may vary. You will know the peanut butter cups are ready when the chocolate is completely set.

NUTRITION FACTS (PER SERVING)

Total Carbohydrates: 4g	Dietary Fiber: 1g	Net Carbs: 3g
Protein: 2g	Total Fat: 10g	Calories: 107

5 minutes **0 minutes**

MINT CHOCOLATE CHIP SHAKE (GF,P)

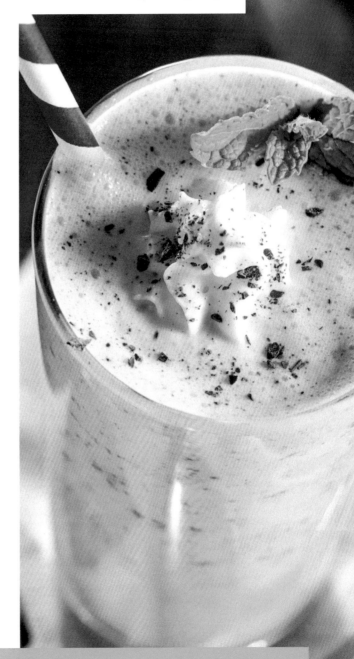

INGREDIENTS

» 1 cup full-fat coconut milk
» 2 tablespoons unsweetened dark chocolate, chopped
» ½ cup mint leaves
» ½ avocado, pitted
» 1 teaspoon pure vanilla extract
» 1 tablespoon sugar substitute (use pure Grade B maple syrup for a paleo version)
» ½ cup ice

DIRECTIONS

1. Add all the ingredients to a high-speed blender and blend until smooth.
2. Enjoy right away.

ADDITIONAL TIP

* The amount of ice you use will determine how thick the shake will be, so adjust according to your liking.

NUTRITION FACTS (PER SERVING)

Total Carbohydrates: 18g	**Dietary Fiber: 7g**	**Net Carbs: 11g**
Protein: 4g	**Total Fat: 21g**	**Calories: 274**

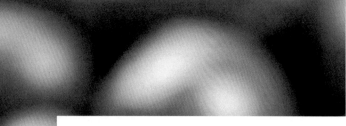

10 minutes (plus time in the fridge)   **5 minutes**   **x8**

CHOCOLATE-COVERED ALMONDS (GF,P)

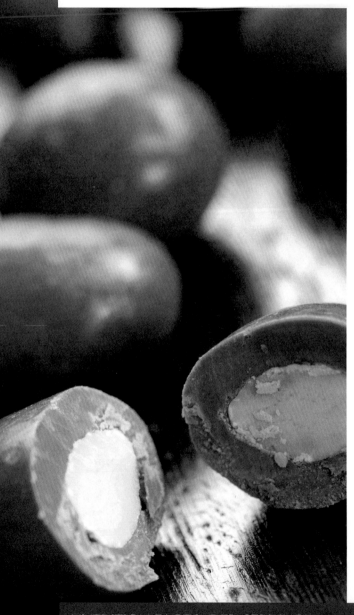

INGREDIENTS

» ¾ cup unsweetened dark chocolate baking chips
» 1½ cups whole raw almonds
» 1 teaspoon pure vanilla extract
» Pinch of sea salt

DIRECTIONS

1. Line a baking sheet with parchment paper and add the chocolate chips to a stockpot over low heat with the vanilla extract.
2. Stir the chocolate until melted.
3. Add the almonds to the stockpot with the melted chocolate and stir until the almonds are coated.
4. Place the almonds onto the lined baking sheet.
5. Sprinkle with salt and set in the fridge for at least 30 minutes before serving.

ADDITIONAL TIP

* Feel free to add a pinch of ground cinnamon to the chocolate mixture for added flavor.

NUTRITION FACTS (PER SERVING)

Total Carbohydrates: 7g	**Dietary Fiber: 4g**	**Net Carbs: 3g**
Protein: 4g	**Total Fat: 15g**	**Calories: 183**

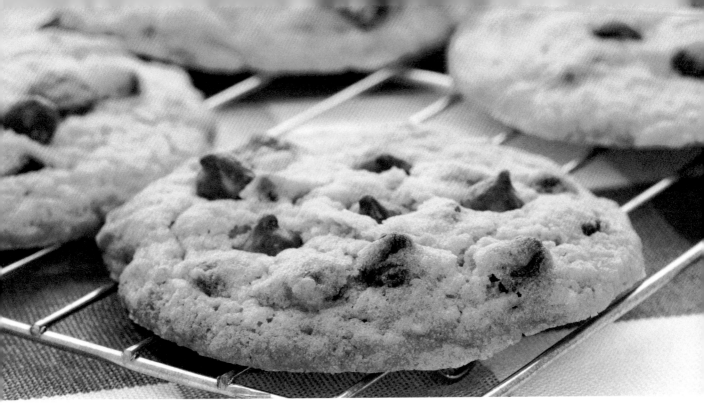

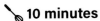 **10 minutes**   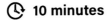 **10 minutes**   **x18**

INGREDIENTS

- » 1 cup unsweetened almond butter
- » ½ cup sugar substitute (use pure Grade B maple syrup for a paleo version)
- » ¼ cup unsweetened dark chocolate baking chips
- » 1 egg
- » 1 teaspoon baking soda
- » 1 teaspoon pure vanilla extract
- » Pinch of sea salt

DIRECTIONS

1. Preheat the oven to 350ºF and line a baking sheet with parchment paper.
2. Add the almond butter, egg, sugar substitute, and vanilla to a large mixing bowl and stir well.
3. Add in the remaining ingredients and stir.
4. Drop the dough by 1-inch rounds onto the baking sheet and bake for 10 minutes or until the edges are brown and lightly crispy.

ADDITIONAL TIP

* Feel free to swap the almond butter out for the nut butter of your choice.

NUTRITION FACTS (PER SERVING)

Total Carbohydrates: 10g	**Dietary Fiber: 1g**	**Net Carbs: 9g**
Protein: 3g	**Total Fat: 10g**	**Calories: 137**

SNICKERDOODLE BITES (GF)

🥄 **10 minutes**   🕐 **0 minutes**   👤 **x12**

INGREDIENTS

» 1 cup unsweetened peanut butter (use almond butter for a paleo version)

» ¼ cup sugar substitute (use pure Grade B maple syrup for a paleo version)

» ¼ cup unsweetened dark chocolate baking chips

» 3 tablespoons coconut flour

» 2 tablespoons unsweetened almond milk

» 1 teaspoon ground cinnamon

» 1 teaspoon pure vanilla extract

» Pinch of sea salt

DIRECTIONS

1. Line a baking sheet with parchment paper.
2. Add all the ingredients to a mixing bowl and mix well.
3. Set in the fridge for 30 minutes.
4. Remove from the fridge and roll into 12 bite-sized balls and place on the lined baking sheet. Set in the fridge for another hour before serving.
5. Store leftovers in the fridge.

ADDITIONAL TIP

* You can use almond butter instead of peanut butter if you desire. You can also roll the bites in unsweetened raw cocoa powder before setting them in the fridge as well.

NUTRITION FACTS (PER SERVING)

Total Carbohydrates: 12g	**Dietary Fiber: 3g**	**Net Carbs: 9g**
Protein: 7g	**Total Fat: 14g**	**Calories: 194**

YOU MAY ALSO LIKE

Please visit the below link for other books by the author

http://ketojane.com/books

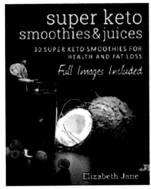
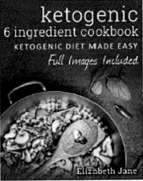
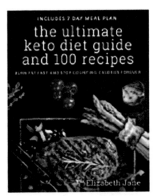

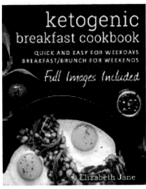
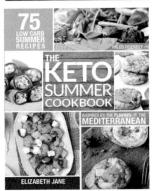
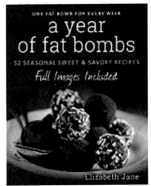

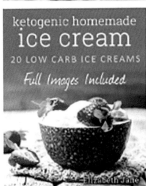
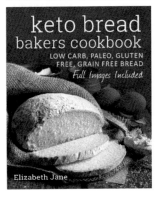
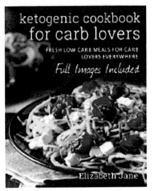

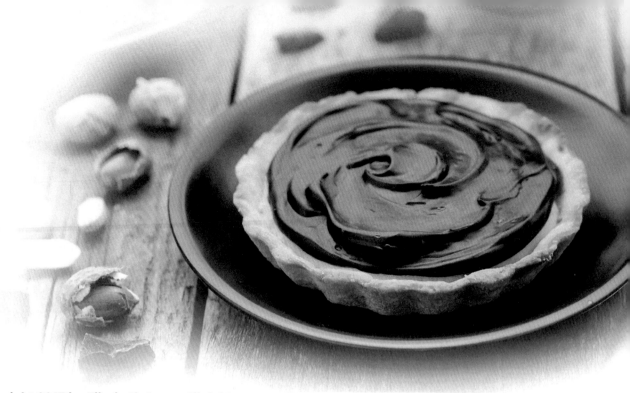

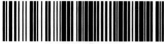

10473511R00024